I0775219

Title: Acid Alkaline Diet Cookbook 2024: Healthy and Nutritious Recipes to Balance Your Body, Embrace Wellness and Energise Your Life and live longer.

By

Linda Compton

COPYRIGHT © (2023)
Except for brief quotations included in critical reviews and certain other noncommercial uses allowed by copyright law, no part of this publication may be reproduced, distributed, or transmitted in any form or by any means, including photocopying, recording, or other electronic or mechanical methods, without the publisher's prior written permission.
I have taken every precaution to guarantee that the information provided is accurate. But the material in this book is provided "as is" with no implied or explicit warranty. Both the publisher and the author disclaim all liability for any harm resulting from this

Table of Contents

Introduction

Welcome to the exciting world of the acid alkaline diet! In this chapter, we will delve into the fundamental principles of the acid alkaline diet, exploring how it can positively impact your health and well-being. We will also provide an overview of the delicious and nutritious recipes that await you in this cookbook, designed to support your journey towards a more balanced and vibrant lifestyle. Get ready to embark on a culinary adventure that not only tantalises your taste buds but also nourishes your body from the inside out. Let's discover the power of the acid alkaline diet together!

What is the acid alkaline diet?

The acid alkaline diet is based on the concept that certain foods can affect the acidity or alkalinity (pH level) of the body. Proponents of this diet believe that by consuming a balanced ratio of acidic and alkaline foods, you can optimise your body's pH levels, promoting better health and reducing the risk of various diseases.

According to the acid alkaline diet philosophy, acidic foods such as meat, dairy, refined sugar, and processed foods can lead to an overly acidic environment in the body, potentially contributing to inflammation, digestive issues, and other health concerns. In contrast, alkaline-forming foods like fruits, vegetables, nuts, and legumes are believed to help counteract excess acidity and create a more alkaline state within the body, potentially supporting overall wellness.

While the scientific evidence supporting the specific health claims of the acid alkaline diet is limited, focusing on a diet rich in fruits, vegetables, and whole foods can undoubtedly have positive effects on overall health and well-being. As with any dietary approach, it's essential to consider individual nutritional needs and consult with a healthcare professional before making significant changes to your diet.

Benefits of following an acid alkaline diet

Proponents of the acid alkaline diet suggest that it may offer several potential benefits, including:

1. **Improved Digestive Health**: The emphasis on consuming alkaline-forming foods such as fruits and vegetables may support a healthy digestive system and help maintain a balanced pH level in the body.

2. **Increased Energy Levels:** Advocates of the diet claim that by reducing the consumption of acidic foods and focusing on alkaline-forming options,

individuals may experience increased energy and vitality.

3. **Reduced Inflammation**: Some believe that following an acid alkaline diet can help reduce inflammation in the body, potentially lowering the risk of certain chronic diseases.

4. **Enhanced Immune Function**: A diet rich in fruits, vegetables, and other alkaline-forming foods may support immune function and overall health.

5. **Weight Management:** The emphasis on whole, nutrient-dense foods may help individuals maintain a healthy weight and support weight management efforts.

It's important to note that the scientific evidence supporting these specific benefits of the acid alkaline diet is limited. However, focusing on a diet that includes a variety of fruits, vegetables, and whole foods can certainly contribute to overall health and well-being. As with any dietary approach, individual needs and medical considerations should be taken into account, and it's best to consult with a healthcare professional before making significant changes to your diet.

Overview of the cookbook

An acid-alkaline diet is based on the idea that certain foods can affect the pH balance (acidity or alkalinity) of the body. The diet promotes consuming a high proportion of alkaline-forming foods such as fruits, vegetables, nuts, seeds, and legumes, while reducing the intake of acid-forming foods like meat, dairy, processed foods, and refined sugar.

Cookbooks related to the acid-alkaline diet often include recipes and meal plans that focus on incorporating alkaline-forming ingredients and achieving a balanced pH level in the body. The recipes may emphasise fresh, whole foods and offer guidance on creating meals that support overall health and well-being.

Chapter One

Understanding pH Balance

Understanding pH balance involves grasping the concept of acidity and alkalinity within substances. In the human body, maintaining a specific pH balance is crucial for various physiological processes. pH is measured on a scale from 0 to 14: lower values signify acidity, higher values indicate alkalinity, and 7 is considered neutral. Different bodily systems have specific pH ranges for optimal function. The body utilises mechanisms like breathing, kidney function, and buffers to regulate and sustain these balances.

Explanation of pH balance and its importance in the body

pH balance, an essential aspect of human physiology, refers to the measurement of acidity or alkalinity within bodily fluids and tissues. This delicate balance profoundly impacts various physiological processes, playing a pivotal role in maintaining optimal health.

The pH scale, ranging from 0 to 14, quantifies the concentration of hydrogen ions in a substance. A pH of 7 denotes neutrality, while values below 7 indicate acidity and above 7 signify alkalinity. In the human body, different systems and organs exhibit specific pH ranges crucial for their proper functioning.

One of the most critical areas where pH balance is imperative is blood. Blood pH typically hovers within a narrow range slightly above neutral, around 7.35 to 7.45. This slight alkalinity is vital for supporting enzymatic reactions and facilitating the transportation of oxygen by haemoglobin. Even a minor deviation from this range can significantly impact enzymatic activity, compromising metabolic processes and disrupting the body's equilibrium, potentially leading to severe health complications.

The body's intricate systems work tirelessly to maintain these precise pH balances. The respiratory system regulates pH through breathing—carbon dioxide, a product of cellular metabolism, can alter blood pH levels. The kidneys play a crucial role in excreting excess acids or bases to maintain the body's pH within the required range. Additionally, various chemical buffer systems exist in bodily fluids to quickly counteract any sudden shifts in pH, preventing drastic changes that could be harmful.

Cellular function heavily relies on optimal pH levels. Enzymes, the catalysts for biochemical reactions, exhibit sensitivity to pH. Any drastic change in pH can disrupt enzyme activity, hindering crucial cellular processes. Moreover, the immune system's ability to ward off pathogens can be affected by pH imbalance, potentially compromising the body's defence mechanisms.

Understanding and maintaining pH balance is fundamental for overall health. It's not merely about avoiding acidity but ensuring that the body's internal environment remains conducive to essential biological processes. Through a concerted effort involving diet, hydration, and lifestyle choices, individuals can actively contribute to sustaining this critical balance for optimal health and well-being.

Impact of acidic and alkaline foods on health

The impact of acidic and alkaline foods on health relates to their potential to influence the body's pH levels and various physiological processes:

Acidic Foods:

1. Bone Health: High intake of acidic foods might lead to calcium loss, potentially affecting bone health.
2. Dental Health: Acidity can erode tooth enamel, contributing to dental issues like cavities.
3. Digestive Discomfort: Acidic foods might trigger acid reflux or digestive discomfort in some individuals.
4. Inflammation: Excessive intake of acidic foods may contribute to inflammation in the body.

1. Bone Health: Alkaline foods could potentially support bone health by reducing calcium loss.
2. Hydration: Many alkaline foods, like fruits and vegetables, are hydrating, aiding overall hydration levels in the body.
3. Reduced Inflammation: Alkaline-rich diets might help reduce inflammation due to their association with antioxidants and phytonutrients.
4. Improved Digestion: Some people report improved digestion and reduced acid reflux symptoms with higher alkaline food intake.

Maintaining a balanced diet that includes a variety of foods from both categories can be beneficial. However, the impact of specific foods can vary among individuals based on their unique physiology and health conditions.

It's important to note that while certain foods are acidic or alkaline in their natural state, their impact on the body's pH after digestion might differ due to complex metabolic processes. The body has mechanisms to regulate pH levels, and overall dietary patterns tend to have a more substantial impact on health than focusing solely on the acidity or alkalinity of individual foods.

How to test your own pH levels

Testing your own pH levels can be done through various methods:

Urine pH Testing:

1. pH Test Strips: Purchase pH test strips from a pharmacy or online. Collect a sample of your urine in a clean container. Dip the test strip into the urine and compare the colour change to the provided chart to determine your pH level.

Saliva pH Testing:

1. pH Test Strips: Similar to urine testing, use pH test strips to collect a sample of saliva in your mouth. Once the strip is moistened, compare the colour change to the provided chart.

Digital pH Metres:

1. Saliva or Urine Testing: Digital pH metres are available for saliva or urine testing. Follow the specific instructions provided with the device to accurately measure your pH levels.

Blood pH Testing:

Testing blood pH requires a medical professional and is typically done in a clinical setting.

- Test your pH levels at the same time each day for consistency.
- Avoid testing immediately after meals, as this can temporarily affect pH levels.
- Keep in mind that pH levels can vary throughout the day due to diet, hydration, and other factors.

Always consult a healthcare professional for proper guidance on interpreting pH test results and to understand how they relate to your overall health and well-being. pH testing at home provides a general indication but might not be as accurate or informative as clinical testing.

Chapter Two

Getting Started with the Acid Alkaline Diet

Getting started with the acid-alkaline diet involves a few key steps:

Understand Acid-Alkaline Principles:

1. Learn about pH Balance: Understand the concept of pH balance in the body and how it relates to health.
2. Identify Acidic and Alkaline Foods: Get familiar with foods categorised as acidic or alkaline and their impact on the body's pH.

Modify Your Diet:

1. Increase Alkaline Foods: Incorporate more alkaline-forming foods such as fruits, vegetables, nuts, seeds, and legumes into your meals.
2. Limit Acidic Foods: Reduce intake of acidic foods like processed foods, meats, dairy, and refined sugars.
3. Stay Hydrated: Drink plenty of water, as it's considered neutral and supports hydration and detoxification.

Monitor and Adapt:

1. pH Testing: Consider using pH test strips to monitor your body's pH levels, though this is optional and not always indicative of overall health.

2. Listen to Your Body: Pay attention to how different foods make you feel. Adjust your diet based on how your body responds.

Seek Guidance:

1. Consult a Professional: If you have health concerns or specific dietary needs, consult a healthcare professional or a registered dietitian before making significant dietary changes.

Gradual Changes:

1. Take Small Steps: Implement changes gradually to allow your body to adapt and make long-term adjustments sustainable.

Focus on Balance:

1. Overall Diet Quality: Remember that balance is key. Focus on an overall balanced and varied diet rather than obsessing over individual food's acidity or alkalinity.

Additional Tips:
Meal Planning: Plan meals that incorporate a variety of alkaline foods.
Educate Yourself: Read books or reputable resources to gain a deeper understanding of the acid-alkaline diet.

Remember, individual responses to dietary changes vary, and what works for one person might not work the same for another. It's important to approach dietary changes with a balanced perspective and consider your unique health circumstances.

Transitioning to an acid-alkaline diet can be a gradual process. Here are some helpful tips:

Gradual Changes:
1. Slow Transition: Start by gradually incorporating more alkaline foods into your meals while reducing acidic ones. Small, sustainable changes over time can be more effective.
2. Focus on Meals: Begin with one meal a day or specific days of the week to introduce alkaline-rich dishes.

Explore Alkaline Foods:

1. Discover New Foods:Experiment with a variety of alkaline foods like fruits, vegetables, nuts, seeds, and legumes. Find recipes that incorporate these ingredients.
2. Replace Acidic Foods:Substitute acidic items with healthier alkaline options. For instance, opt for plant-based proteins instead of animal proteins.

Meal Planning:

1. Plan Ahead: Plan your meals to include a balance of alkaline foods. This can make the transition smoother and more manageable.

2. Batch Cooking: Prepare larger portions of alkaline-based meals to have ready-to-eat options available throughout the week.

1. Stay Hydrated: Drink plenty of water as it supports a more balanced pH and overall health.
2. Reduce Stress: Stress can impact pH levels. Incorporate stress-relieving activities like meditation or exercise into your routine.

Educate Yourself:
1. Learn About Foods: Understand which foods are more alkaline and acidic to make informed choices.
2. Consult Resources: Utilise books, reputable websites, or consult with a dietitian for guidance and recipes.

Listen to Your Body:
1. Monitor Reactions: Pay attention to how your body responds to changes. Adjust your diet based on how you feel.
2. Be Patient: It might take time for your body to adjust to dietary changes. Be patient with yourself during this transition.

Seek Support:
1. Community or Groups: Consider joining online communities or groups where you can get tips, share experiences, and find support from others following similar dietary paths.

Remember, the key is to make sustainable changes that work for your lifestyle and health goals. It's not about a sudden overhaul but about creating a healthier eating pattern over time.

Certainly! Here are some pantry essentials that align with the principles of the acid-alkaline diet:

Alkaline Foods:
1. Fruits: Apples, berries, bananas, lemons, limes, and watermelon.
2. Vegetables: Leafy greens (spinach, kale), broccoli, cauliflower, carrots, bell peppers, and cucumbers.
3. Nuts and Seeds: Almonds, chia seeds, flaxseeds, and pumpkin seeds.
4. Legumes: Lentils, chickpeas, and beans (black beans, kidney beans).

Neutral Foods:
1. Whole Grains: Quinoa, millet, brown rice, and oats.
2. Healthy Oils: Olive oil, avocado oil, and coconut oil.

Acidic Foods (to consume in moderation):
1. Animal Proteins: Limit red meat and opt for leaner sources like chicken or fish.
2. Dairy: Limit dairy products like cheese and milk.

3. Processed Foods: Minimise processed and packaged foods high in sugars and artificial additives.

Others:
1. Herbs and Spices: Turmeric, ginger, garlic, basil, oregano, and cilantro.
2. Apple Cider Vinegar: Considered acidic but often believed to have an alkalizing effect on the body.
3. Filtered Water: Staying hydrated with clean water is crucial for maintaining pH balance.

Tips:
Fresh Produce: Aim for fresh fruits and vegetables as much as possible.
Variety: Include a wide variety of foods from different categories to ensure a balanced diet.
Whole Foods: Opt for whole, unprocessed foods over refined options.

These items can form the basis of a well-rounded acid-alkaline balanced diet. Always consider individual health conditions and consult with a healthcare professional or a registered dietitian before making significant dietary changes.

Meal planning and grocery shopping guide

Meal Planning Tips:
1. Plan Ahead: Set aside time to plan your meals for the week, considering a balance of alkaline foods.

2. Include Variety: Aim for diverse meals with fruits, vegetables, nuts, seeds, and whole grains.

3. Batch Cooking: Prepare larger portions of grains, legumes, or soups that can be used in multiple meals.

4. Balance Your Plate: Ensure each meal includes a mix of protein, healthy fats, carbohydrates, and plenty of veggies.

Grocery Shopping Guide:

1. Fruits and Vegetables: Stock up on a variety of fresh produce, including leafy greens, berries, citrus fruits, broccoli, carrots, and bell peppers.

2. Whole Grains: Purchase quinoa, brown rice, oats, and whole-grain pasta or bread.

3. Legumes: Include lentils, chickpeas, black beans, and other beans for protein sources.

4. Nuts and Seeds: Buy almonds, chia seeds, flaxseeds, and pumpkin seeds for added nutrients.

5. Healthy Oils: Opt for olive oil, avocado oil, and coconut oil.

6. Herbs and Spices: Have turmeric, ginger, garlic, basil, and oregano on hand for flavour.

7. Lean Proteins: If consuming animal proteins, choose lean options like chicken, fish, or turkey in moderation.

8. Filtered Water: Ensure you have ample clean water available for hydration.

Shopping Tips:

1. Stick to Your List: Plan your meals and create a shopping list accordingly to avoid impulse purchases.
2. Shop the Perimeter: Most fresh and whole foods are typically found around the edges of the grocery store.
3. Read Labels: Be mindful of ingredients in packaged items and try to choose minimally processed options.
4. Buy in Bulk: Consider purchasing staple items like grains, nuts, and seeds in bulk to save money.

Additional Considerations:

Flexibility: Be open to trying new recipes and adapting meals based on what's available or on sale at the store.
Preparation: Consider prepping ingredients ahead of time to streamline cooking during busy days.
Health Priorities: Always prioritise your health needs and dietary preferences when planning meals and shopping.

Remember, meal planning and grocery shopping are highly individualised. Customise your approach based on your preferences, dietary requirements, and lifestyle.

Chapter Three

Breakfast Recipes

Delicious and nutritious

Certainly! Here are a few delicious and nutritious breakfast recipes that align with the principles of an acid-alkaline diet:

1. Alkaline Smoothie Bowl:
Ingredients:
  - 1 frozen banana
  - 1 cup mixed berries (strawberries, blueberries, raspberries)
  - 1 handful spinach or kale
  - ½ avocado
  - ½ cup almond milk or coconut water
  - Toppings: Chia seeds, sliced almonds, fresh fruits

Instructions:
  1. Blend the banana, berries, spinach or kale, avocado, and almond milk or coconut water until smooth.
  2. Pour the smoothie into a bowl.
  3. Top with chia seeds, sliced almonds, and fresh fruits.

2. Quinoa Breakfast Bowl:

Ingredients:
  - 1 cup cooked quinoa
  - Sliced fresh fruits (such as mangoes, berries, or bananas)
  - ¼ cup nuts (almonds, walnuts)
  - 1 tablespoon honey or maple syrup (optional)
  - Cinnamon for flavour

Instructions:
  1. In a bowl, layer cooked quinoa as the base.
  2. Top with sliced fruits and nuts.
  3. Drizzle honey or maple syrup if desired and sprinkle with cinnamon.

3. Avocado Toast with Poached Eggs:
Ingredients:
  - Whole-grain bread slices
  - Ripe avocado
  - Eggs
  - Salt, pepper, and chilli flakes (optional)
  - Lemon juice

Instructions:
  1. Toast the whole-grain bread slices.
  2. Mash ripe avocado and spread it on the toast.
  3. Poach or fry eggs and place them on top of the avocado.
  4. Season with salt, pepper, chilli flakes, and a squeeze of lemon juice.

4. Chia Seed Pudding:
Ingredients:

- ¼ cup chia seeds
- 1 cup almond milk or coconut milk
- Fresh fruits for topping
- Optional: Honey or maple syrup for sweetness

Instructions:
  1. Mix chia seeds and almond milk in a bowl. Let it sit for 10-15 minutes, stirring occasionally until it thickens.
  2. Once thickened, pour into serving cups and refrigerate for a few hours or overnight.
  3. Top with fresh fruits before serving.

These recipes offer a mix of nutrients, flavours, and textures, perfect for a nutritious start to your day while aligning with an acid-alkaline diet. Adjust ingredients and toppings based on personal preferences and dietary needs.

breakfast recipes to kickstart your day

Absolutely! Here are energising breakfast recipes to kickstart your day:

  1. Greek Yoghourt Parfait:
Ingredients:
  - Greek yoghourt
  - Mixed berries (strawberries, blueberries, raspberries)
  - Granola
  - Honey or maple syrup (optional)

Instructions:

1. Layer Greek yoghurt, mixed berries, and granola in a glass or bowl.

2. Drizzle honey or maple syrup for added sweetness if desired.

2. Vegetable Omelette:
Ingredients:

- Eggs

- Chopped vegetables (bell peppers, spinach, tomatoes)

- Olive oil

- Salt, pepper, and herbs (like basil or oregano)

Instructions:

1. Whisk eggs in a bowl and season with salt, pepper, and herbs.

2. Sauté chopped vegetables in olive oil until slightly tender.

3. Pour the whisked eggs over the vegetables and cook until set to make an omelette.

3. Quinoa Fruit Salad:
Ingredients:

- Cooked quinoa

- Assorted fruits (mangoes, kiwi, pineapple, oranges)

- Mint leaves for garnish

- Lemon or lime juice

Instructions:

1. Mix cooked quinoa with chopped fruits in a bowl.

2. Squeeze fresh lemon or lime juice for a tangy flavour.

3. Garnish with mint leaves before serving.

4. Spinach and Mushroom Breakfast Wrap:
Ingredients:
- Whole-grain wrap or tortilla
- Sautéed spinach and mushrooms
- Scrambled eggs or tofu (for a vegan option)
- Avocado slices
- Salsa or hot sauce (optional)

Instructions:
1. Lay out the wrap and add scrambled eggs or tofu, sautéed spinach and mushrooms, avocado slices, and salsa or hot sauce.

2. Roll up the wrap and enjoy.

5. Overnight Oats:
Ingredients:
- Rolled oats
- Chia seeds
- Almond milk or any preferred milk
- Sliced bananas, nuts, or berries for topping

Instructions:
1. Mix rolled oats, chia seeds, and almond milk in a jar or bowl.

2. Refrigerate overnight.

3. Top with sliced bananas, nuts, or berries before eating.

These breakfast options offer a balance of nutrients, providing energy and a flavorful start to your day! Adjust ingredients to suit your preferences and dietary needs.

Certainly! Here are some examples of morning meals rich in alkaline foods:

1. Green Smoothie:
Ingredients:
  - Spinach or kale
  - Cucumber
  - Celery
  - Green apple
  - Lemon juice
  - Coconut water or almond milk

Instructions:
  1. Blend spinach or kale, cucumber, celery, green apple, a splash of lemon juice, and your choice of liquid until smooth.
  2. Enjoy a refreshing and nutrient-packed green smoothie.

2. Chia Seed Breakfast Pudding:
Ingredients:
  - Chia seeds

- Almond milk or coconut milk
- Sliced almonds
- Berries (blueberries, strawberries)
- Optional: Maple syrup or honey for sweetness

Instructions:
1. Mix chia seeds and almond milk in a jar or bowl and refrigerate overnight.
2. In the morning, top with sliced almonds and fresh berries. Add a drizzle of maple syrup or honey if desired.

3. Alkaline Fruit Salad:
Ingredients:
- Sliced mangoes
- Pineapple chunks
- Kiwi slices
- Fresh berries (blueberries, raspberries)
- Lime juice

Instructions:
1. Mix all the sliced fruits in a bowl.
2. Squeeze fresh lime juice over the fruit salad for a citrusy kick.

4. Avocado Toast with Alkaline Vegetables:
Ingredients:
- Whole-grain toast
- Mashed avocado
- Sliced cucumber
- Tomato slices
- Sprouts (alfalfa or broccoli sprouts)

- Lemon juice
- Optional: Sprinkle of sesame seeds

Instructions:
   1. Spread mashed avocado on whole-grain toast.
   2. Layer with sliced cucumber, tomato, and sprouts.
   3. Squeeze fresh lemon juice on top and add sesame seeds if desired.

5. Quinoa Breakfast Bowl with Alkaline Veggies:
Ingredients:
   - Cooked quinoa
   - Steamed broccoli florets
   - Sautéed spinach
   - Sliced bell peppers
   - Toasted pumpkin seeds
   - Optional: Drizzle of olive oil

Instructions:
   1. Mix cooked quinoa with steamed broccoli, sautéed spinach, sliced bell peppers, and toasted pumpkin seeds in a bowl.
   2. Add a drizzle of olive oil for extra flavour if desired.

These morning meals incorporate alkaline-rich ingredients like leafy greens, fruits, and vegetables, providing a nutritious start to your day. Adjust ingredients and portions to suit your taste preferences and dietary needs.

Absolutely! Here are some quick and easy breakfast ideas perfect for busy mornings:

1. Overnight Oats:
Ingredients:
  - Rolled oats
  - Chia seeds
  - Almond milk or any preferred milk
  - Sliced bananas, nuts, or berries for topping

Instructions:
  1. Mix rolled oats, chia seeds, and almond milk in a jar or bowl the night before.
  2. Refrigerate overnight and top with sliced bananas, nuts, or berries in the morning.
Ready-to-eat without any cooking!

2. Whole Grain Toast with Nut Butter:
Ingredients:
  - Whole-grain bread
  - Nut butter (peanut, almond, or cashew)
  - Sliced fruits (banana, apple)

Instructions:
  1. Toast whole-grain bread and spread nut butter on top.
  2. Add sliced fruits for a quick, balanced breakfast.

3. Yogurt Parfait:
Ingredients:
  - Greek yoghourt

- Granola or muesli
- Mixed berries or sliced fruits
- Optional: Honey or maple syrup for sweetness

Instructions:
1. Layer Greek yoghurt, granola, and mixed berries in a jar or bowl.
2. Drizzle with honey or maple syrup if desired.

4. Fruit Smoothie:
Ingredients:
- Frozen mixed berries
- Banana
- Spinach or kale
- Almond milk or coconut water
- Optional: Protein powder or nut butter for added protein

Instructions:
1. Blend frozen berries, banana, spinach or kale, almond milk or coconut water, and optional protein powder or nut butter until smooth.

5. Egg Muffin Cups:
Ingredients:
- Eggs
- Chopped vegetables (bell peppers, spinach)
- Shredded cheese (optional)
- Salt, pepper, and herbs

Instructions:

1. Whisk eggs and mix in chopped vegetables, cheese, salt, pepper, and herbs.

2. Pour into greased muffin cups and bake until set for a quick grab-and-go breakfast.

These breakfast ideas are simple, require minimal preparation, and can be customised with your favourite toppings or ingredients. They're perfect for hectic mornings when time is limited.

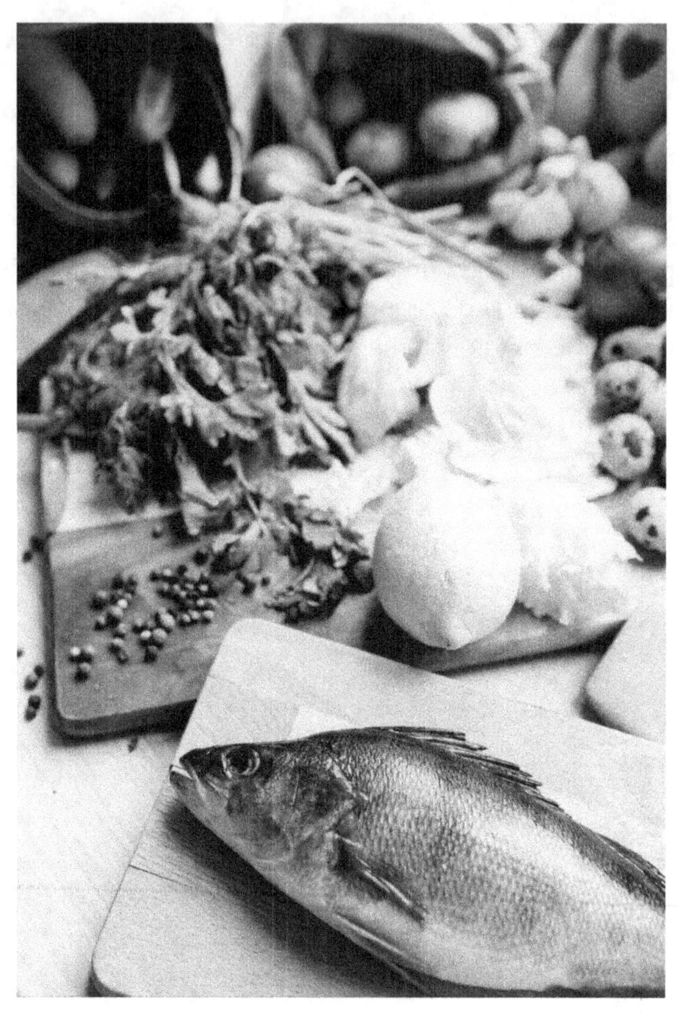

Chapter Four

Lunch and Dinner Ideas

Absolutely! For flavorful and satisfying lunches and dinners within the Acid Alkaline Diet Cookbook, consider dishes like:

Lunch Ideas:

1. Quinoa Salad with Roasted Vegetables: A colourful mix of quinoa, roasted bell peppers, cherry tomatoes, and spinach, tossed in a light citrus vinaigrette.
2. Stuffed Bell Peppers: Bell peppers stuffed with a blend of quinoa, black beans, corn, and spices, baked until tender.
3. Chickpea Salad Wrap: Whole grain wrap filled with a refreshing mix of chickpeas, diced cucumbers, red onions, and a tahini dressing.
4. Veggie Stir-Fry with Brown Rice: A medley of colourful vegetables stir-fried in a light sesame oil sauce, served over brown rice.
5. Mediterranean Veggie Bowl: A bowl featuring roasted vegetables, olives, hummus, and a sprinkle of feta cheese on a bed of greens.

1. Baked Lemon Herb Tilapia: Tilapia fillets seasoned with herbs and baked with lemon slices, served alongside steamed broccoli and quinoa.
2. Vegetable Curry: A flavorful mix of vegetables simmered in a coconut milk-based curry sauce, served with brown rice or quinoa.
3. Portobello Mushroom Burgers: Grilled portobello mushrooms marinated in balsamic vinegar, served on whole grain buns with avocado, lettuce, and tomato.
4. Zucchini Noodles with Pesto: Zucchini noodles tossed in homemade basil pesto and topped with cherry tomatoes and pine nuts.
5. Lentil and Vegetable Soup: A hearty soup made with lentils, carrots, celery, and tomatoes, seasoned with herbs and spices.

These dishes focus on vibrant flavours, nutrient-rich ingredients, and a balance between alkaline-promoting foods to create both satisfying and healthy lunch and dinner options.

Flavorful and satisfying lunch and dinner recipes

Absolutely, here are a few flavorful and satisfying recipes perfect for lunch and dinner:

Lunch Recipes:

1. Mango Avocado Quinoa Salad:
Combine cooked quinoa, diced mango, avocado
chunks, red onion, cilantro, and a lime vinaigrette.
Serve chilled.

2. Greek Salad with Grilled Chicken:
  - Mix together cucumber, cherry tomatoes, red
onion, Kalamata olives, feta cheese, and grilled
chicken strips. Dress with olive oil, lemon juice, and
oregano.

3. Sweet Potato and Black Bean Burrito Bowl:
  - Roast sweet potato cubes and toss with black
beans, corn, chopped lettuce, salsa, and a dollop of
Greek yoghurt. Serve over brown rice or quinoa.

Dinner Recipes:

1. Lemon Herb Grilled Salmon:
  - Marinate salmon fillets in a mix of lemon juice,
olive oil, garlic, and herbs. Grill until cooked through
and serve with roasted vegetables.

2. Vegetable Stir-Fry with Tofu:**
  - Stir-fry bell peppers, broccoli, snap peas, and
tofu in a mix of soy sauce, ginger, and garlic. Serve
over brown rice or noodles.

3. Eggplant Parmesan:

- Bread eggplant slices, bake until crispy, then layer them with marinara sauce and mozzarella cheese. Bake until bubbly and golden brown.

These recipes offer a mix of flavours, textures, and nutrients, making them both satisfying and delicious for lunch or dinner.

Incorporating alkaline foods into your main meals

Absolutely! Here are ways to incorporate alkaline foods into your main meals:

1. Load Up on Vegetables:
Salads: Start meals with alkaline-rich salads filled with leafy greens, cucumbers, bell peppers, tomatoes, and radishes.
Stir-Fries: Prepare vegetable stir-fries using alkaline veggies like broccoli, spinach, kale, bok choy, and bell peppers.

2. Choose Alkaline Grains:
Opt for grains like quinoa, millet, and amaranth instead of processed grains. Use these as bases for dishes like pilafs, salads, or alongside main courses.

3. Incorporate Alkaline Proteins:
Legumes: Include beans, lentils, and chickpeas in soups, stews, salads, or as the main protein in dishes.

Tofu or Tempeh: Use tofu or tempeh in stir-fries, curries, or marinated and grilled dishes.

4. Healthy Fats and Oils:
Avocado: Enjoy avocado in salads, wraps, or as a topping for various dishes.
Nuts and Seeds: Sprinkle nuts and seeds like almonds, chia seeds, or pumpkin seeds over salads or incorporate them into dishes for added nutrients.

5. Herbal Infusions and Beverages:
Herbal Teas: Choose herbal teas like chamomile, ginger, or peppermint that have alkaline properties.
Green Smoothies: Blend alkaline fruits like kiwi, avocado, and berries with leafy greens for a nutritious alkaline-rich beverage.

6. Alkaline Seasonings and Herbs:
Herbs: Use alkaline herbs like basil, parsley, cilantro, and dill to add flavour to dishes.
Spices: Incorporate alkaline spices such as turmeric, ginger, and cinnamon into your cooking.

By focusing on these categories of alkaline foods, you can create balanced and nutritious meals while maintaining the alkaline balance in your diet.

One-pot meals and meal prep options for convenience

Absolutely, one-pot meals and meal prep options can significantly ease the cooking process while ensuring convenience and efficiency. Here are some ideas:

One-Pot Meals:

1. Vegetable Quinoa Pilaf: Cook quinoa in vegetable broth with sautéed onions, garlic, and your choice of alkaline vegetables like bell peppers, spinach, and zucchini. Season with herbs and spices for flavour.

2. Lentil Soup/Stew: Combine lentils, alkaline vegetables (carrots, celery, kale), tomatoes, and vegetable broth in one pot. Add herbs and spices for taste. Let it simmer until the lentils are tender.

3. Chickpea Curry: Sauté onions, garlic, and ginger. Add chickpeas, diced tomatoes, coconut milk, and alkaline veggies like cauliflower and spinach. Simmer until the flavours meld.

Meal Prep Options:

1. Grain Bowls: Cook a batch of quinoa, brown rice, or farro. Portion into containers and add cooked alkaline vegetables, beans, or grilled tofu. Store dressings separately to maintain freshness.

2. Roasted Vegetables: Roast a variety of alkaline vegetables (bell peppers, broccoli, carrots) with olive oil, salt, and pepper. Use them as sides, add to salads, or as toppings for bowls throughout the week.

3. Pre-Cut and Marinated Proteins: Pre-cut tofu, tempeh, or chicken. Marinate them in alkaline-friendly sauces or herbs. When ready to eat, quickly cook or bake for a speedy and healthy meal.

These options allow for quick and easy preparation while ensuring you have nutritious and alkaline-friendly meals ready to go, whether it's a one-pot creation or a pre-prepped component waiting to be assembled.

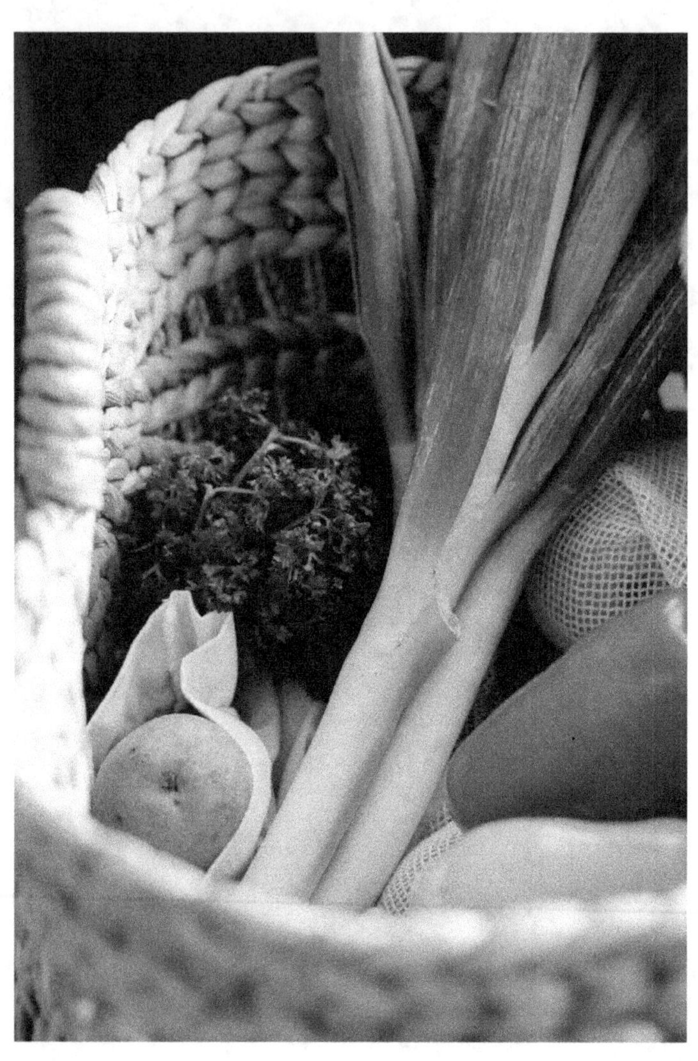

Chapter Five

Snacks and Sides

Snacks:

1. Almonds or Almond Butter: A handful of almonds or a spoonful of almond butter is a great alkaline-rich snack.

2. Hummus with Veggie Sticks: Enjoy hummus (made with chickpeas, tahini, lemon, and garlic) with sliced alkaline veggies like carrots, cucumber, and bell peppers.

3. Chia Seed Pudding: Combine chia seeds with almond milk, a touch of maple syrup, and vanilla extract. Let it sit in the fridge until it thickens into a pudding-like consistency. Top with alkaline fruits like berries.

4. Rice Cakes with Avocado: Spread mashed avocado on rice cakes for a quick and satisfying alkaline snack.

Side Dishes:

1. Roasted Root Vegetables: Roast alkaline root veggies such as beets, carrots, and sweet potatoes with olive oil and herbs for a flavorful side dish.

2. Steamed Greens: Steam alkaline greens like kale, spinach, or Swiss chard. Add a splash of lemon juice or a drizzle of olive oil for extra flavour.

3. Cauliflower Rice: Pulse cauliflower in a food processor to create rice-like grains. Sauté with garlic, onions, and alkaline spices for a healthy alternative to traditional rice.

4. Quinoa Salad: Prepare a refreshing salad with cooked quinoa mixed with diced alkaline vegetables, herbs, and a lemon vinaigrette.

These snacks and side dishes not only provide alkaline-rich options but also offer a variety of flavours and textures to complement your meals or curb hunger between them.

Healthy and alkaline snack options

Absolutely, here are some healthy and alkaline snack options:

1. Cucumber Slices with Hummus: Enjoy cucumber slices dipped in hummus, a combination that offers hydrating properties from the cucumber and alkalinity from the chickpeas in the hummus.

2. Almond Butter on Rice Cakes: Spread almond butter on rice cakes for a satisfying snack that

combines the alkalinity of almonds with the neutral pH of rice cakes.

3. Green Smoothies: Blend alkaline ingredients like spinach, kale, avocado, and a splash of almond milk or coconut water for a nutrient-packed, alkaline-rich snack.

4. Mixed Nuts: Snack on a handful of almonds, walnuts, or cashews, as these nuts tend to be more alkaline-forming.

5. Chia Seed Pudding: Create chia seed pudding by mixing chia seeds with almond milk and a touch of maple syrup or vanilla extract. Top with alkaline fruits like berries for added flavour.

6. Bell Pepper Strips with Guacamole: Slice bell peppers into strips and pair them with homemade guacamole made from avocado, lime juice, garlic, and cilantro for a delicious and alkaline-rich snack.

7. Kale Chips: Bake kale leaves tossed with a bit of olive oil and sea salt until crispy for a crunchy and nutritious alkaline snack alternative to regular chips.

These snacks provide a mix of nutrients, flavours, and textures while being aligned with an alkaline diet to help maintain a balanced pH in the body.

Side dishes to accompany your meals

Certainly! Here are some side dish options that complement various meals:

1. Steamed Broccoli with Garlic Butter:
   - Steam fresh broccoli until tender-crisp, then toss it in a light garlic-infused olive oil or butter for added flavour.

2. Quinoa Pilaf:
   - Cook quinoa with sautéed onions, garlic, and herbs. Add diced alkaline vegetables like bell peppers, carrots, and peas for a flavorful and nutritious side.

3. Roasted Root Vegetables:
   - Roast a medley of root vegetables such as sweet potatoes, beets, and carrots with olive oil, herbs, and a touch of balsamic vinegar for a caramelised and savoury side.

4. Sautéed Spinach with Garlic:
   - Quickly sauté spinach with minced garlic in olive oil until wilted. Finish with a squeeze of lemon juice for brightness.

5. Cauliflower Mash:
   - Steam or boil cauliflower until tender, then mash it with a bit of almond milk, garlic, and herbs for a lighter alternative to mashed potatoes.

6. Green Salad with Avocado Dressing:

- Toss a mix of leafy greens, cucumber, tomatoes, and radishes with a creamy avocado-based dressing made from mashed avocado, lemon juice, and a touch of olive oil.

7. Grilled Asparagus:
   - Grill asparagus spears with a drizzle of olive oil, salt, and pepper until they develop a slight char for a simple yet elegant side.

These side dishes offer a variety of flavours and textures, enhancing the main course while ensuring a balanced and nutritious meal.

Portable snack ideas for on-the-go

Absolutely! Here are some portable snack ideas that are perfect for on-the-go situations:

1. Trail Mix: Create your mix with almonds, walnuts, pumpkin seeds, dried fruits like apricots or raisins, and a sprinkle of unsweetened coconut flakes for a balanced, energy-boosting snack.

2. Fruit and Nut Bars: Opt for homemade or store-bought bars made with simple ingredients like dates, nuts, seeds, and dried fruits without added sugars or preservatives for a convenient and nutritious snack.

3. Whole Fruit: Grab fruits like apples, bananas, oranges, or berries that are easy to carry and consume without any preparation needed.

4. Veggie Sticks with Hummus: Portion out carrot sticks, cucumber slices, or bell pepper strips and pair them with individual servings of hummus for a refreshing and crunchy snack.

5. Rice Cakes with Nut Butter: Spread almond or peanut butter on rice cakes and pack them for a quick and satisfying snack that's easy to transport.

6. Greek Yogurt Parfait: Pre-portion Greek yoghurt into a portable container and top it with nuts, seeds, and a drizzle of honey or a few slices of alkaline fruits like kiwi or berries.

7. Hard-Boiled Eggs: Prepare hard-boiled eggs in advance and carry them in a container with a sprinkle of salt and pepper for a protein-rich snack.

8. Roasted Chickpeas: Roast chickpeas with spices like paprika, cumin, and garlic powder until crispy for a crunchy and protein-packed snack.

These portable snack options are convenient, nutritious, and can easily be taken along wherever your day takes you.

Chapter Six

Desserts and Treats

Absolutely! Here are some dessert and treat ideas that align with an alkaline diet:

1. Fruit Salad with Mint: Combine alkaline fruits like berries, kiwi, and pineapple. Add a touch of fresh mint and a squeeze of lime juice for a refreshing dessert.

2. Almond Date Balls: Blend dates, almonds, and a hint of vanilla extract in a food processor. Roll the mixture into balls and coat them with shredded coconut for a naturally sweet treat.

3. Baked Apples with Cinnamon: Core apples and sprinkle them with cinnamon. Bake until tender for a warm, comforting dessert without added sugars.

4. Chia Seed Pudding with Berries: Create a chia seed pudding by mixing chia seeds, almond milk, and a touch of maple syrup. Top with alkaline berries like blueberries or raspberries for a delightful treat.

5. Frozen Banana Bites: Slice bananas, dip them in melted dark chocolate, and freeze for a satisfying and indulgent dessert option.

6. Coconut Yogurt Parfait: Layer coconut yoghurt with chopped alkaline fruits and a sprinkle of nuts or seeds for a creamy, dairy-free dessert.

7. Avocado Chocolate Mousse: Blend ripe avocado, cocoa powder, a touch of honey or maple syrup, and a splash of almond milk until smooth. Chill for a few hours for a rich and creamy dessert.

8. Baked Pears with Almonds: Slice pears and bake them with a sprinkle of almonds, cinnamon, and a drizzle of honey until tender for a comforting and lightly sweet dessert.

These desserts and treats offer a variety of flavours and textures while adhering to an alkaline diet, allowing you to enjoy something sweet while maintaining a balanced pH in the body.

Indulgent yet alkaline-friendly dessert recipes

Absolutely, here are some indulgent yet alkaline-friendly dessert recipes:

1. Raw Chocolate Avocado Mousse:
   - Blend ripe avocados, cocoa powder, a touch of maple syrup or honey, and a splash of almond milk until smooth. Chill before serving for a creamy and decadent mousse.

2. Almond Butter Banana Bites:
  - Slice bananas into rounds, spread almond
butter between two slices, and freeze them for a
sweet and creamy treat.

3. Berry Coconut Popsicles:
  - Blend alkaline fruits like strawberries,
blueberries, or raspberries with coconut water. Pour
the mixture into popsicle moulds and freeze for a
refreshing dessert.

4. Date and Nut Energy Balls:
  - Blend dates, almonds, coconut flakes, and a
hint of vanilla extract in a food processor. Roll the
mixture into balls and coat them with crushed nuts
for a sweet and satisfying snack.

5. Chia Seed Chocolate Pudding:
  - Mix chia seeds, cocoa powder, almond milk, and
a touch of sweetener (like maple syrup or agave).
Let it sit in the fridge until it thickens into a rich
pudding.

6. Baked Stuffed Apples:
  - Core apples and fill the centre with a mixture of
chopped nuts, dried fruits, cinnamon, and a drizzle
of honey. Bake until tender for a warm and
delightful dessert.

7. Coconut Almond Bliss Balls:
  - Blend coconut flakes, almonds, a bit of coconut
oil, and a touch of honey in a food processor. Roll

the mixture into balls and coat them with more coconut flakes for a tropical treat.

These desserts maintain an indulgent feel while incorporating alkaline-friendly ingredients, offering a balance between sweetness and nutritional value.

Healthy alternatives to satisfy your sweet tooth

Absolutely, here are some healthy alternatives to satisfy your sweet tooth:

1. Fruit Salad or Fruit Kabobs: Enjoy a variety of fresh alkaline fruits like berries, melons, kiwi, and pineapple for a naturally sweet treat without added sugars.

2. Frozen Grapes: Freeze grapes for a refreshing and sweet snack that mimics the texture of sorbet without any added sugar.

3. Yogurt Parfait with Berries: Layer Greek yoghurt with alkaline berries and a sprinkle of nuts or seeds for a creamy, satisfying, and naturally sweet dessert.

4. Dark Chocolate: Indulge in a small portion of high-quality dark chocolate (70% or higher cocoa content) as it contains less sugar and is rich in antioxidants.

5. Banana "Ice Cream": Blend frozen bananas until creamy for a dairy-free, naturally sweetened "ice cream" alternative. Add cocoa powder or berries for flavour variations.

6. Baked Cinnamon Apples: Slice apples, sprinkle with cinnamon, and bake until tender for a warm and comforting dessert without added sugars.

7. Homemade Smoothie: Blend almond milk, alkaline fruits, and a touch of honey or dates for a naturally sweetened, nutrient-packed beverage.

8. Coconut Date Rolls: Blend dates and shredded coconut in a food processor, roll them into bite-sized balls, and chill. These provide a natural sweetness from dates and a satisfying texture from coconut.

These alternatives offer sweetness from natural sources, providing a healthier option to satisfy your sweet cravings while aligning with an alkaline-friendly diet.

Tips for incorporating alkaline ingredients into baking

Certainly! Here are some tips for incorporating alkaline ingredients into baking:

1. Use Alkaline Flour Alternatives:

- Substitute traditional flours with alkaline alternatives like spelt flour, buckwheat flour, or almond flour. These options provide a higher alkaline content compared to wheat flour.

2. Incorporate Alkaline Sweeteners:
   - Opt for natural alkaline sweeteners such as maple syrup, agave nectar, or coconut sugar instead of refined sugars. These alternatives add sweetness while being less acidic.

3. Add Alkaline-Rich Fruits and Nuts:
   - Include alkaline-rich ingredients like bananas, apples, berries, and almonds in your baked goods. They not only contribute to the alkalinity but also add moisture and flavour.

4. Use Alkaline-Friendly Leavening Agents:
   - Choose baking powder or baking soda as leavening agents, which are alkaline, rather than yeast, which can be more acidic.

5. Include Alkaline Spices and Herbs:
   - Incorporate alkaline spices and herbs like cinnamon, ginger, and parsley into your recipes to enhance flavours while promoting alkalinity.

6. Balance Acidic Ingredients:
   - If using acidic ingredients like citrus juices or vinegar, consider balancing them with alkaline ingredients or buffering agents like baking soda to neutralise their acidity.

7. Experiment and Adjust Recipes:
   - Gradually experiment with substituting ingredients in your favourite recipes. Adjust quantities and ratios to find the right balance of alkaline ingredients while maintaining taste and texture.

8. Alkaline Additions in Frostings and Toppings:
   - Consider using coconut-based or almond-based frostings or toppings instead of those based on acidic ingredients like cream cheese or sour cream.

By incorporating these tips, you can adapt your baking recipes to include more alkaline ingredients, promoting a healthier balance while still enjoying delicious baked goods.

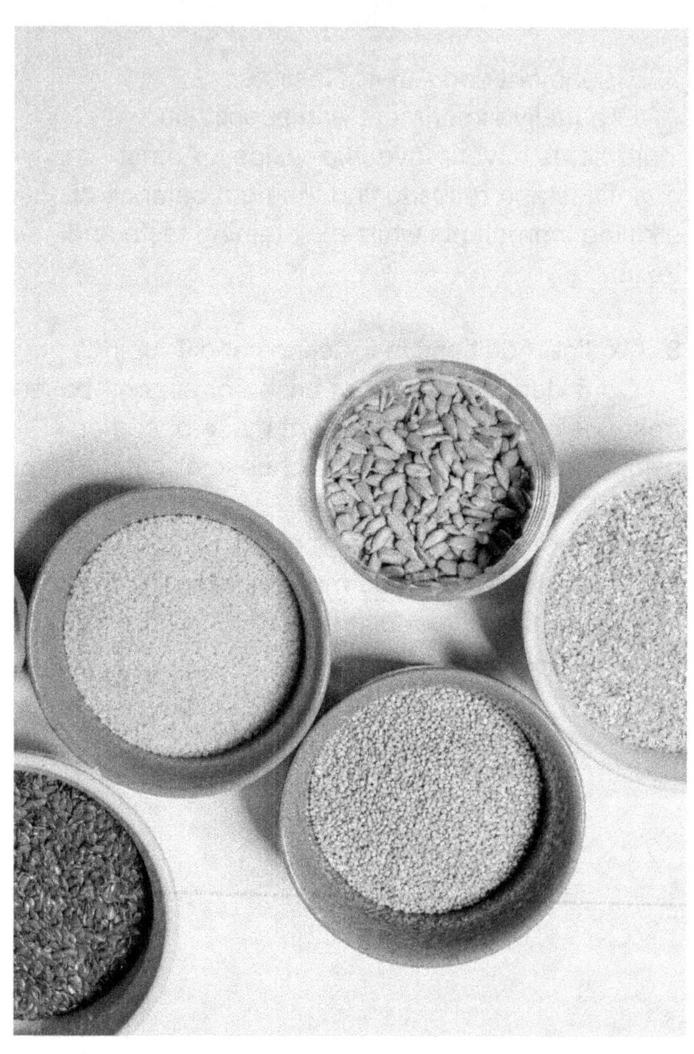

Chapter Seven

Beverages and Smoothies

Certainly! Here are some alkaline-friendly beverage and smoothie ideas:

Beverage Options:

1. Alkaline Water: Drinking water with a higher pH level can help maintain alkalinity in the body. Consider alkaline water sourced from natural minerals or a water ioniser.

2. Herbal Teas: Chamomile, ginger, peppermint, and dandelion teas are herbal options that can contribute to alkalinity in the body.

3. Fresh Green Juices: Juices made from alkaline vegetables like kale, spinach, cucumber, and celery provide nutrients and support the alkaline balance.

4. Coconut Water: Natural coconut water is alkaline-forming and can be a refreshing and hydrating beverage choice.

Smoothie Ideas:

1. Green Smoothie: Blend alkaline-rich leafy greens (spinach, kale), cucumber, celery, a splash of lemon juice, and an alkaline fruit like green apple for a nutritious and alkaline smoothie.

2. Berry Blast Smoothie: Combine alkaline berries (blueberries, raspberries), a banana, almond milk, a spoonful of almond butter, and a handful of spinach for a sweet and satisfying smoothie.

3. Tropical Paradise Smoothie: Blend pineapple, mango, coconut water, spinach, and a scoop of chia seeds for a flavorful and alkaline-rich tropical beverage.

4. Cucumber Avocado Smoothie: Mix cucumber, avocado, lime juice, a handful of spinach, and coconut water for a creamy and refreshing alkaline smoothie.

5. Almond Butter Banana Smoothie: Blend banana, almond butter, almond milk, a sprinkle of cinnamon, and a date for a creamy and naturally sweet alkaline beverage.

These beverage and smoothie options not only taste delicious but also help maintain an alkaline balance in the body by incorporating alkaline-forming ingredients.

Refreshing and hydrating drink recipes

Absolutely! Here are some refreshing and hydrating drink recipes perfect for maintaining hydration:

1. Cucumber Mint Infused Water:
   - Combine thinly sliced cucumber and fresh mint leaves with water. Let it infuse for a few hours in the fridge for a refreshing and hydrating drink.

2. Citrus Spa Water:
   - Slice lemons, limes, and oranges and add them to a pitcher of water with a few sprigs of fresh rosemary or basil for a citrus-infused hydrating drink.

3. Watermelon Cooler:
   - Blend chunks of watermelon with a splash of lime juice and a handful of mint leaves. Strain the mixture and serve over ice for a revitalising beverage.

4. Iced Herbal Teas:
   - Brew herbal teas like chamomile, hibiscus, or peppermint, let them cool, and serve over ice for a calming and hydrating drink.

5. Coconut Cucumber Refresher:
   - Mix coconut water with cucumber slices and a squeeze of lime for a hydrating and electrolyte-rich drink.

6. Green Tea with Citrus:

- Brew green tea and let it cool. Add slices of lemon or orange for a citrusy twist. Serve it chilled for a refreshing and antioxidant-packed beverage.

7. Sparkling Berry Splash:
  - Muddle fresh berries (such as strawberries, raspberries, or blueberries) in a glass, add sparkling water, and a squeeze of lime for a fizzy and hydrating drink.

These refreshing and hydrating drink recipes provide a flavorful way to stay hydrated while enjoying the benefits of natural ingredients.

Alkaline smoothie ideas for a nutrient boost

Absolutely! Here are some alkaline smoothie ideas that offer a nutrient boost:

1. Green Goddess Smoothie:
- Ingredients: Spinach, kale, cucumber, green apple, a squeeze of lemon juice, and coconut water. Blend for a nutrient-packed, alkaline-rich green smoothie.

2. Berry Blast Smoothie:
- Ingredients: Mixed berries (blueberries, strawberries, raspberries), a handful of spinach, almond milk, a spoonful of almond butter, and a sprinkle of chia seeds for a delicious and nutritious drink.

3. Tropical Green Smoothie:
- Ingredients: Pineapple, mango, spinach, coconut water, and a scoop of hemp seeds for a tropical and nutrient-dense alkaline beverage.

4. Avocado Banana Smoothie:
- Ingredients: Avocado, banana, almond milk, a handful of kale, and a spoonful of honey or maple syrup for a creamy and satisfying alkaline smoothie.

5. Citrus Spinach Smoothie:
- Ingredients: Oranges, pineapple, spinach, coconut water, and a small piece of ginger for a zesty and refreshing nutrient boost.

6. Almond Butter Green Smoothie:
- Ingredients: Almond butter, mixed greens (kale, spinach), cucumber, a splash of lemon juice, and coconut water for a creamy and alkaline-rich drink.

7. Kiwi Coconut Smoothie:
- Ingredients: Kiwi, coconut milk or coconut water, a handful of greens (such as spinach or kale), and a sprinkle of flaxseeds for a tangy and nutritious smoothie.

These smoothie recipes offer a variety of flavours while incorporating alkaline-rich ingredients, providing a nutrient-packed boost to your day.

Certainly! While it's important to note that the effectiveness of homemade alkaline water may vary compared to commercially produced alkaline water, here are a couple of DIY recipes you can try:

1. Lemon and Baking Soda Alkaline Water:
Ingredients:
  - 1 litre of purified or filtered water
  - 1 lemon
  - 1/2 teaspoon of baking soda

Instructions:
  1. Squeeze the juice of one lemon into the water.
  2. Add 1/2 teaspoon of baking soda and stir until it dissolves.
  3. Let the mixture sit for a few minutes before drinking. The lemon and baking soda combination may create a more alkaline environment in the water.

2. Cucumber and Mint Alkaline Water:
Ingredients:
  - 1 litre of purified or filtered water
  - 1 cucumber
  - A handful of fresh mint leaves

Instructions:
  1. Slice the cucumber and place the slices in the water.
  2. Add the fresh mint leaves to the water.

3. Let the water sit for a few hours or overnight in the refrigerator to allow the cucumber and mint to infuse into the water, potentially increasing its alkalinity.

These homemade recipes may slightly increase the pH of the water due to the presence of alkaline-promoting ingredients like lemon, baking soda, cucumber, or mint. However, their effectiveness might not match the level of alkalinity achieved through specialised equipment used in commercial alkaline water production. Always consider consulting a healthcare professional before making significant changes to your water consumption habits.

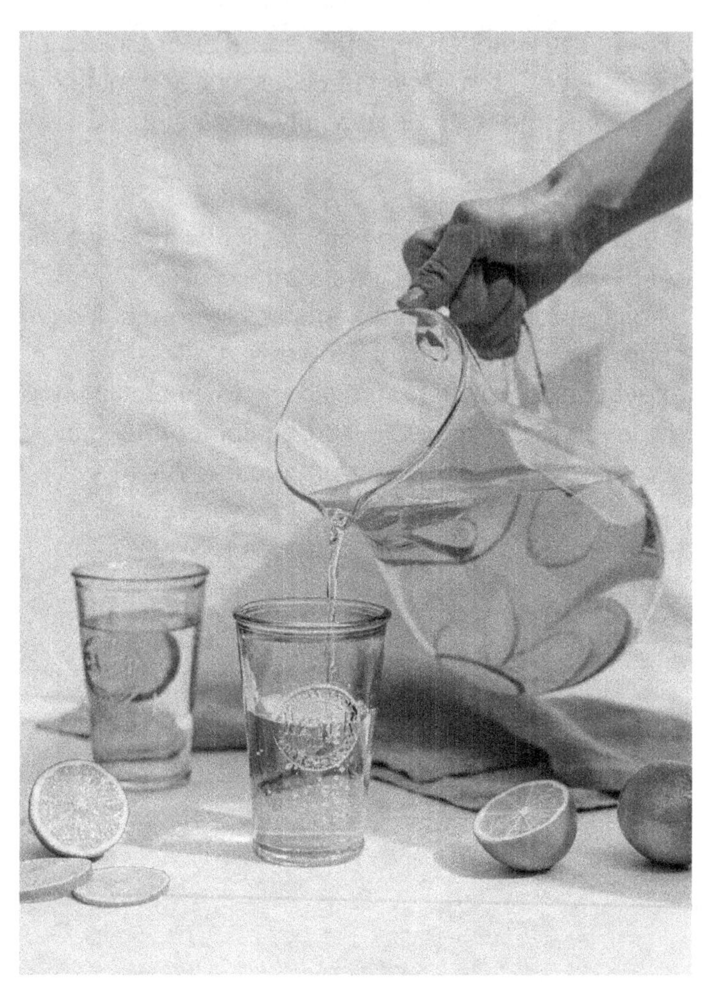

Chapter Eight

Special Occasions and Entertaining

Absolutely, special occasions and entertaining provide opportunities to create memorable experiences with food, drinks, and ambiance. Here are ideas for special occasions and entertaining while keeping an alkaline-friendly focus:

1. Alkaline Appetisers:
   - Offer platters of fresh vegetable crudites with hummus or guacamole, nuts and seeds, or whole-grain crackers with almond-based spreads.

2. Alkaline-Friendly Salads:
   - Prepare colourful salads with leafy greens, alkaline vegetables like bell peppers, tomatoes, and cucumbers, topped with nuts, seeds, and a light vinaigrette.

3. Main Courses with Alkaline Ingredients:
   - Serve grilled or roasted alkaline-rich vegetables, such as asparagus, broccoli, and cauliflower. Consider offering options like grilled fish or tofu as protein choices.

4. Desserts with a Twist:
   - Create fruit-based desserts like fruit salads, fruit skewers, or mixed berry parfaits with coconut

cream for a naturally sweet yet alkaline-friendly ending.

5. Mocktails and Refreshments:
   - Prepare alkaline-infused beverages like cucumber or citrus-infused water, herbal teas, or sparkling water with berries for refreshing non-alcoholic options.

6. Presentation and Ambiance:
   - Enhance the atmosphere with fresh flowers, candles, and soft lighting. Consider using natural decor elements to create an inviting setting.

7. Flexibility and Communication:
   - Communicate with guests about the alkaline-friendly menu options, ensuring everyone can enjoy the meal while being informed about the choices available.

8. Customization:
   - Offer a "build-your-own" salad or bowl station where guests can assemble their meals using alkaline-friendly ingredients, catering to individual preferences.

By incorporating alkaline-rich foods and drinks into your special occasions and entertaining, you can create a diverse and enjoyable experience for your guests while aligning with a health-conscious approach.

Alkaline recipes for special events and gatherings

Absolutely, here's a selection of alkaline recipes perfect for special events and gatherings:

Appetisers:

1. Stuffed Bell Peppers: Fill bell peppers with a mix of quinoa, black beans, tomatoes, and spices. Bake until tender for a satisfying appetiser.

2. Zucchini Rolls with Hummus: Thinly slice zucchini lengthwise, spread with hummus, and roll them up for a light and flavorful starter.

Salads:

1. Mango Avocado Salad: Combine diced mango, avocado, red onion, cilantro, and lime juice for a refreshing and vibrant salad.

2. Cauliflower Tabouli: Pulse cauliflower in a food processor until rice-like, mix with chopped parsley, tomatoes, cucumber, and lemon juice for a twist on a classic tabouli salad.

Main Courses:

1. Grilled Lemon Herb Chicken: Marinate chicken in a blend of lemon juice, olive oil, garlic, and herbs. Grill until cooked through for a flavorful main dish.

2. Quinoa and Roasted Vegetable Platter: Serve a colourful platter of roasted vegetables alongside a quinoa pilaf for a wholesome and hearty main course.

Desserts:

1. Chia Seed Pudding Parfaits: Layer chia seed pudding made with almond milk and sweetened with a touch of maple syrup with fresh berries and nuts for a delicious dessert.

2. Baked Apples with Cinnamon: Core apples, sprinkle with cinnamon and a bit of coconut sugar, and bake until tender for a warm and comforting sweet treat.

Beverages:

1. Herbal Infused Waters: Offer pitchers of water infused with cucumber, mint, and lemon slices for a refreshing and hydrating drink option.

2. Green Tea Lemonade: Combine green tea with freshly squeezed lemon juice and a touch of honey for a revitalising and alkaline-friendly beverage.

These recipes incorporate alkaline-rich ingredients while offering a variety of flavours and textures, making them ideal for special events and gatherings.

Certainly! Here are some hosting tips for serving alkaline-friendly dishes at gatherings or events:

Plan a Diverse Menu:

- Create a well-rounded menu that includes a variety of alkaline-rich foods like fresh vegetables, fruits, whole grains, legumes, nuts, and seeds to cater to different tastes and preferences.

Label or Describe Dishes:

- Provide labels or descriptions for each dish, mentioning the alkaline ingredients used, especially for guests who might be following specific dietary preferences or restrictions.

Offer Balanced Options:
- Ensure a balance between raw and cooked alkaline foods to provide different textures and flavours. Raw salads, cooked vegetable dishes, and protein options like grilled fish or tofu can add variety.

Prepare Customizable Meals:
- Consider setting up a "build-your-own" bowl or salad station where guests can create their meals, incorporating various alkaline ingredients based on their preferences.

Highlight Alkaline Beverages:

- Showcase alkaline-infused beverages like herbal teas, infused waters, or fresh fruit juices as refreshing drink options throughout the event.

Accommodate Dietary Needs:
- Take note of any dietary needs or preferences your guests might have (like gluten-free or vegan) and ensure there are options available that align with those requirements.

Presentation Matters:
- Present the dishes in an appealing manner by using colourful plates, garnishes, and serving bowls to make the alkaline-friendly dishes visually enticing.

Communicate with Guests:
- Let your guests know in advance about the alkaline-friendly nature of the menu, providing an overview of what they can expect and ensuring they feel informed and comfortable.

By incorporating these hosting tips, you can offer a delightful and enjoyable experience while serving alkaline-friendly dishes, catering to your guests' dietary needs and preferences.

How to enjoy the acid alkaline diet while dining out

Enjoying the acid-alkaline diet while dining out can be manageable with a few strategies:

1. Research and Choose Wisely:

- Before dining out, look up the menu online or call the restaurant to inquire about their offerings. Opt for places that offer a variety of fresh vegetables, salads, and lean protein options.

2. Customization is Key:
- Don't hesitate to ask for modifications or substitutions to make your meal more alkaline-friendly. For example, request a side of steamed vegetables instead of fries or a salad instead of bread.

3. Focus on Vegetables and Greens:
- Look for dishes centred around alkaline vegetables like salads, roasted or steamed vegetables, and vegetable-based soups.

4. Protein Choices:
- Choose lean proteins like grilled chicken, fish, tofu, or beans as they tend to be more alkaline-forming.

5. Be Mindful of Sauces and Dressings:
- Ask for sauces, dressings, and condiments on the side. This way, you have control over how much you use, minimising intake of acidic components.

6. Avoid Overly Processed or Fried Foods:
- Steer clear of heavily processed or fried items as they often contain ingredients that may lean more towards the acidic side.

7. Hydration Matters:
- Opt for water or herbal teas instead of sugary or caffeinated drinks, promoting hydration and supporting the alkaline balance in your body.

8. Portion Control:
- Be mindful of portion sizes. Even if the dish is generally alkaline-friendly, excessive amounts might still affect the body's pH balance.

9. Mindful Eating:
- Enjoy your meal mindfully, focusing on the taste and quality of the food. Eating slowly can also aid digestion and allow your body to process nutrients more effectively.

10. Be Flexible and Enjoy the Experience:
- While aiming for alkaline-friendly options is ideal, it's also essential to enjoy dining out as a social experience. Try to strike a balance between enjoying the occasion and making healthier choices.

With these tips, you can navigate dining out while adhering to an acid-alkaline diet, making more informed choices to support your dietary preferences.

Chapter Nine

Maintenance and Sustainability

Maintaining an acid-alkaline balanced diet and ensuring its sustainability involves a few key principles:

1. Consistency in Food Choices:
- Strive for consistency in incorporating alkaline-rich foods into your daily meals. Aim for a balanced intake of fruits, vegetables, nuts, seeds, and whole grains to support the body's pH balance.

2. Education and Awareness:
- Continuously educate yourself about alkaline-forming foods and acidic foods to make informed choices. Stay updated on new research and information about maintaining pH balance.

3. Balanced Approach:
- While aiming for an alkaline diet, also focus on overall balance and variety in your meals. Balance alkaline foods with other essential nutrients for a holistic approach to health.

4. Lifestyle Adaptations:
- Incorporate lifestyle factors beyond diet, like stress management, exercise, and adequate sleep,

as they also contribute to overall well-being and a balanced pH.

5. Sustainable Choices:
- Choose sustainably sourced and organic options whenever possible. This supports not only your health but also the environment.

6. Gradual Changes:
- Implement dietary changes gradually, allowing your body to adjust and making it more sustainable in the long run.

7. Flexibility and Enjoyment:
- Maintain flexibility in your diet. While focusing on alkaline-rich foods, allow yourself occasional treats or foods that may be more acidic in nature, especially during special occasions or social gatherings.

8. Regular Monitoring:
- Monitor your body's responses to dietary changes. Keep a journal or note how you feel after consuming certain foods to better understand their effects on your body's pH balance.

9. Consulting Professionals:
- Consider consulting a registered dietitian or healthcare professional who specialises in nutrition to get personalised guidance and ensure you're meeting your nutritional needs while maintaining pH balance.

By adopting a balanced and informed approach, integrating alkaline-friendly foods into your lifestyle, and considering overall wellness, you can sustain an acid-alkaline balanced diet effectively for improved health and vitality.

Strategies for maintaining a balanced pH in the long term

Maintaining a balanced pH in the long term involves several strategies:

1. Alkaline-Rich Diet:
- Consistently consume a diet rich in alkaline-forming foods such as fruits, vegetables, nuts, seeds, legumes, and whole grains. These help maintain a balanced pH in the body.

2. Hydration:
- Stay well-hydrated by drinking plenty of water, which can support the body's natural pH balance.

3. Limit Acidic Foods:
- Reduce the consumption of highly acidic foods and beverages like processed foods, refined sugars, alcohol, and excessive caffeine, which can potentially disrupt pH balance.

4. Stress Management:

- Practise stress-reducing techniques like meditation, yoga, or deep breathing exercises. Chronic stress can affect the body's pH levels.

5. Regular Exercise:
- Engage in regular physical activity. Exercise promotes circulation, oxygenation, and overall health, potentially aiding in pH balance.

6. Monitor Body Responses:
- Pay attention to how your body responds to different foods. Keep a journal to track how certain foods impact your energy levels, digestion, and overall well-being.

7. pH Testing:
- Periodically check your body's pH levels through testing methods recommended by healthcare professionals. This can offer insights into your body's acidity or alkalinity.

8. Balanced Lifestyle Habits:
- Prioritise adequate sleep, maintain a healthy weight, and avoid smoking or excessive alcohol consumption, as these factors can influence pH balance.

9. Regular Health Check-Ups:
- Schedule regular check-ups with healthcare professionals to assess overall health, including the body's pH balance, if necessary.

10. Consult Professionals:
- Seek advice from registered dietitians,
nutritionists, or healthcare providers who specialise
in pH balance or nutrition for personalised guidance
and recommendations.

By incorporating these strategies into your lifestyle,
you can maintain a more balanced pH in the long
term, supporting overall health and well-being.

Overcoming challenges and sticking to the diet

Sticking to an acid-alkaline balanced diet can pose
challenges, but there are ways to overcome them:

1. Plan and Prepare:
- Plan your meals in advance, create shopping lists,
and prepare ingredients ahead of time to avoid
last-minute decisions that might stray from the diet.

2. Educate Yourself:
- Understand the principles behind the diet.
Knowing why certain foods are chosen can
motivate you to stick with the plan.

3. Gradual Changes:
- Make gradual changes to your diet rather than
attempting an abrupt overhaul. Small, sustainable
steps lead to lasting habits.

4. Variety and Creativity:

- Incorporate a wide variety of alkaline foods to keep meals interesting and enjoyable. Experiment with new recipes and cooking methods to prevent monotony.

5. Flexibility and Moderation:
- Allow some flexibility in your diet. It's okay to occasionally indulge in less alkaline foods, especially during social events, as long as it's in moderation.

6. Social Support:
- Seek support from family, friends, or online communities following similar dietary patterns. Sharing experiences and tips can be encouraging.

7. Mindful Eating:
- Practise mindful eating by paying attention to hunger cues, savouring flavours, and eating slowly. This helps in making conscious food choices aligned with the diet.

8. Addressing Cravings:
- Find alkaline-friendly alternatives to satisfy cravings. For example, choose fruit instead of sugary snacks or herbal teas instead of caffeinated beverages.

9. Accountability and Tracking:
- Keep a food journal or use apps to track meals, noting how you feel after consuming different foods. It helps identify patterns and stay accountable.

10. Be Kind to Yourself:
- Understand that dietary changes take time and might not always be perfect. Be patient and compassionate with yourself through the process.

Remember, the goal is progress, not perfection. Celebrate small victories, stay focused on the benefits of the diet, and be patient with yourself as you navigate and adapt to a new way of eating.

Additional resources and support for continued success

Certainly! Here are some additional resources and support avenues that can aid in continued success with an acid-alkaline balanced diet:

1. Books and Literature:
- Explore books and literature on acid-alkaline diets. Authors like Dr. Robert O. Young and Shelley Redford Young have written extensively on the subject.

2. Registered Dietitians or Nutritionists:
- Consult with a registered dietitian or nutritionist specialised in pH-balanced diets. They can provide personalised guidance and support.

3. Online Communities and Forums:

- Join online communities, forums, or social media groups dedicated to alkaline diets. These platforms offer support, advice, and shared experiences.

4. Apps and Tools:
- Use mobile apps or online tools designed for tracking dietary intake, monitoring pH levels, or accessing alkaline-friendly recipes.

5. Cooking Classes or Workshops:
- Attend cooking classes or workshops focused on alkaline-friendly cooking. Learning new recipes and cooking techniques can make the diet more enjoyable.

6. Wellness Retreats or Seminars:
- Consider attending wellness retreats, seminars, or workshops that cover holistic approaches to health, including pH-balanced diets.

7. Healthcare Professionals:
- Regularly consult with healthcare professionals knowledgeable about pH balance and nutrition to ensure you're on track with your dietary goals.

8. Educational Websites and Articles:
- Explore reputable websites, blogs, or articles by health experts specialising in alkaline diets. These platforms often provide valuable information and resources.

9. Podcasts and Webinars:

- Listen to podcasts or attend webinars featuring experts discussing pH balance, alkaline diets, and related health topics.

10. Personal Support Network:
- Lean on your personal support network—friends, family, or colleagues—for encouragement and accountability in maintaining your dietary choices.

Having access to these resources and support systems can provide ongoing motivation, education, and assistance in maintaining a successful acid-alkaline balanced diet for improved health and well-being.

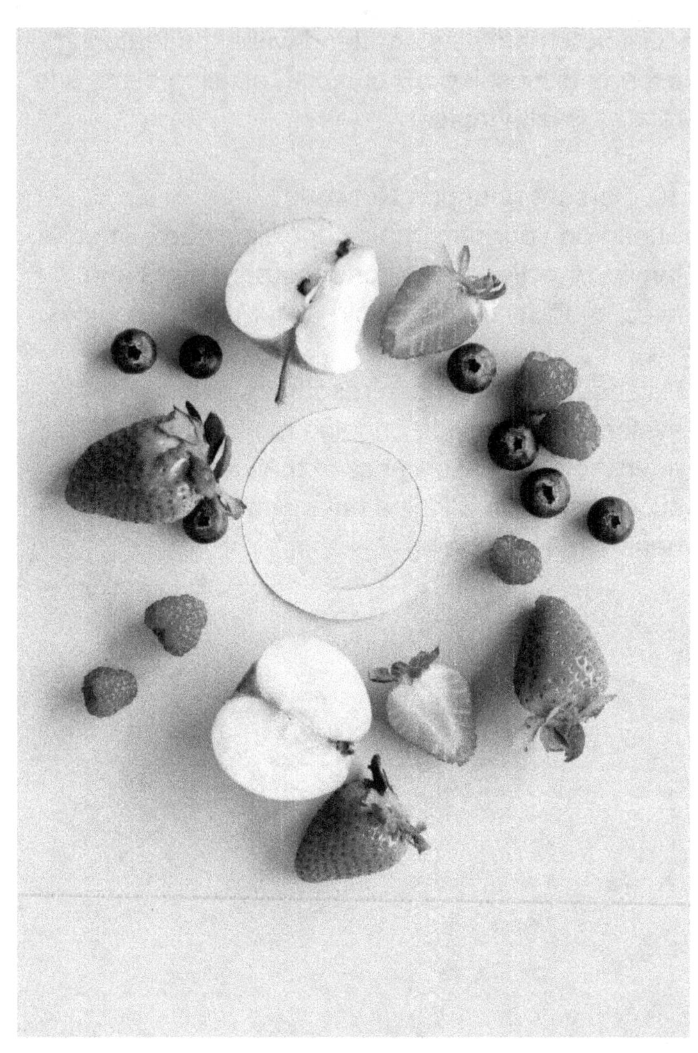

Conclusion

In conclusion, adopting an acid-alkaline balanced diet involves prioritising alkaline-rich foods while minimising acidic choices. This dietary approach aims to promote overall health, enhance energy levels, and support the body's natural balance.

Through a focus on fruits, vegetables, nuts, seeds, legumes, and whole grains, individuals can create a more alkaline environment within the body. Additionally, incorporating lifestyle factors such as stress management, regular exercise, and adequate hydration contributes to a more balanced pH.

While challenges may arise when adhering to this dietary lifestyle, various strategies—such as planning, education, flexibility, and seeking support—can help overcome these obstacles and sustain long-term success.

Remember, the key lies in gradual changes, consistency, and finding a personalised approach that works for your body and lifestyle. Strive for balance, stay informed, and seek guidance from healthcare professionals or experts specialised in pH-balanced diets to ensure a holistic and sustainable approach to health and wellness.

Ultimately, by making informed dietary choices, staying mindful of food intake, and embracing a well-rounded lifestyle, individuals can achieve a more balanced pH and reap the benefits of an acid-alkaline balanced diet for improved overall health and vitality.

Recap of key points

Of course! Here's a recap of the key points regarding an acid-alkaline balanced diet:

1. Alkaline-Rich Foods: Prioritise fruits, vegetables, nuts, seeds, legumes, and whole grains to create a more alkaline environment in the body.

2. Minimise Acidic Foods: Reduce intake of highly processed foods, refined sugars, alcohol, and excessive caffeine to maintain a balanced pH.

3. Lifestyle Factors: Incorporate stress management, regular exercise, hydration, and adequate sleep to support the body's natural pH balance.

4. Education and Awareness: Understand the principles behind the diet and its effects on the body's pH levels to make informed dietary choices.

5. Flexibility and Moderation: Allow some flexibility in the diet while aiming for alkaline-rich foods.

Occasional indulgences in less alkaline foods are acceptable in moderation.

6. Support and Resources: Seek support from registered dietitians, online communities, educational resources, and healthcare professionals specialising in pH-balanced diets.

7. Consistency and Gradual Changes: Strive for gradual dietary changes, maintain consistency in food choices, and embrace a balanced lifestyle for sustainable success.

Remember, an acid-alkaline balanced diet isn't about perfection but about making conscious choices to support overall health and well-being. Incorporating these principles gradually into your lifestyle can lead to lasting benefits.

Encouragement and motivation for embracing the acid alkaline lifestyle

Embracing an acid-alkaline balanced lifestyle is a journey towards improved health and vitality. Here's some encouragement and motivation for this path:

1. Increased Energy and Vitality: By prioritising alkaline-rich foods, you're providing your body with essential nutrients, potentially leading to increased energy levels and overall vitality.

2. Holistic Well-being: This lifestyle isn't just about what you eat; it's about supporting your body's natural balance. Embracing this approach promotes holistic well-being, addressing both physical and mental health.

3. Long-term Health Benefits: Research suggests that an alkaline-rich diet may contribute to reducing inflammation, supporting bone health, and aiding in weight management, fostering long-term health benefits.

4. Personalised Wellness: Every step you take towards an alkaline lifestyle is a step towards personalised wellness. It's about finding what works best for your body and health goals.

5. Small Changes, Big Impact: Even small changes towards alkaline-friendly choices can make a significant impact on your overall health. Celebrate every positive choice you make along the way.

6. Empowerment through Knowledge: Educating yourself about the effects of different foods on your body's pH balance empowers you to make informed choices, taking charge of your health.

7. Feeling Good Inside Out: As you embrace this lifestyle, you might notice improvements in how you feel—more energy, improved digestion, clearer skin—reflecting the positive changes happening inside your body.

8. Progress over Perfection: Remember, it's about progress, not perfection. Embrace the journey, allow yourself flexibility, and be proud of every step you take towards a more balanced lifestyle.

9. You're Worth the Investment: Prioritising your health and well-being through an acid-alkaline balanced lifestyle is a valuable investment in yourself. You deserve to feel your best.

10. Support and Community: You're not alone on this journey. Seek support from others, share experiences, and celebrate successes together as you navigate this lifestyle change.

Embrace this journey with positivity, patience, and a sense of empowerment. Every choice you make towards a more balanced pH contributes to a healthier and happier you.

Looking ahead to a healthier future

Looking ahead to a healthier future means embracing the possibilities of improved well-being, vitality, and longevity. Here's to envisioning the path forward:

1. Optimal Health and Vitality: Embrace the potential of feeling your best—energised, vibrant, and balanced—by prioritising an acid-alkaline balanced diet and lifestyle.

2. Building Resilience: Nourish your body with alkaline-rich foods, setting the stage for a resilient immune system, improved digestion, and enhanced overall health.

3. Long-Term Wellness: Visualise the long-term benefits—an overall sense of wellness, reduced inflammation, strengthened bones, and a healthier weight—through sustained commitment to a balanced pH.

4. Empowerment through Choice: Recognize the power within you to make positive choices daily, shaping your health destiny and creating a future filled with vitality and wellness.

5. Holistic Self-Care: Embrace a holistic approach to self-care, understanding that what you eat, how you move, and your mental well-being collectively contribute to a healthier future.

6. Inspiring Others: By leading by example, you have the opportunity to inspire others in your circle—friends, family, and community—to prioritise their health and well-being.

7. Continued Growth and Learning: Embrace the journey of continued growth and learning about your body, nutrition, and well-being, staying open to new information and discoveries.

8. Adaptability and Balance: Embrace adaptability in your journey. Balance is key, and allowing flexibility while maintaining focus on your health goals ensures sustainable progress.

9. Celebrating Milestones: Acknowledge and celebrate milestones—big or small—as you progress on your journey towards a healthier future. Every positive step matters.

10. Gratitude and Mindfulness: Practise gratitude and mindfulness, appreciating your body's ability to adapt, thrive, and heal as you nourish it with alkaline-rich foods and a balanced lifestyle.

Looking ahead to a healthier future means envisioning a life filled with vitality, wellness, and a profound sense of well-being. Every step you take today paves the way for a brighter, healthier tomorrow.

www.ingramcontent.com/pod-product-compliance
Lightning Source LLC
Chambersburg PA
CBHW060954260726
48661CB00005B/1880